● **About the Autl**

David Boyle is the author of a range of books about social change, history, politics and he regularly writes about the future of volunteering, cities and business. Co-founder of Time Banking UK, David Boyle also helped found the London Time Bank and has been instrumental in developing co-production in Britain as a critical element of public service reform. He is a fellow of the New Economics Foundation (NEF), has been a candidate for Parliament and currently sits on the federal policy committee of the Liberal Democrats.

Sarah Bird is the CEO of Timebanking UK and has over 10 years of experience within the timebanking field, from having originally set up and run a time bank, to becoming a consultant and project manager within Timebanking UK. Sarah continues to develop partnerships and networks across the country with the vision of co-produced timebanking being present in every town and city in the country.

GIVE AND TAKE

HOW TIMEBANKING IS TRANSFORMING HEALTHCARE

David Boyle and Sarah Bird

 Timebanking UK

First edition published in paperback in Great Britain in 2014 by
Timebanking UK
The Exchange, Brick Row
Stroud, Gloucester
GL5 1DF
+44 (0)1453 750952
info@timebanks.co.uk
http://www.timebanking.org

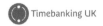
A CIP catalogue record for this book
is available from the British Library.

ISBN: 978-0-9930579-0-8 (print)
ISBN: 978-0-9930579-1-5 (ePub)

 Timebanking UK

Registered charity number: 1101204
Company number: 4502783

Timebanking UK supports The Forest Stewardship Council [FSC], the leading
international forest certification organization. All Timebanking UK
book titles are printed on FSC certified paper.

Project Managed by EDDEPRO Services,
Kingsbridge, TQ7 1HG
Cover design and art direction by Kathryn Evans-Prosser at www.kathrynep.com
Typeset by Tetragon, London

Printed and bound in Great Britain by TJ International,
Padstow PL28 8RW

Contents

✿ Introduction

"There is a clearly stated resolve by NHS policy makers 'to tap into the enthusiasm and energy of patients, the public and local communities' with the aim of making a culture of involvement"

Department Of Health

Imagine that health professionals had the time to make everyone feel valued and cared for personally. Imagine there was an infinite resource to provide the kind of informal care that keeps people healthy. Imagine there was enough time. That was the background to one of the strangest pieces of research ever undertaken in the NHS.

Dr Mike Dixon, once chair of the GP's lobby group the NHS Alliance, was the brave doctor who ran one of the most controversial, yet revealing, experiments ever conducted in a GP surgery. He made a series of complementary therapies available in his clinic in the village of Cullompton in Devon, and then measured the results.

But it was more than just the usual therapies. The experiment happened to coincide with the visit of a local healer, the wife of a judge, who arrived at his surgery and asked him for a job. Dixon was fascinated, and especially with the possibilities for research. What is interesting about healers is that they don't use pills or needles. It is just them, their hands, and their relationship with the patient that counts.

It became clear quite quickly that the healer was making a difference. She was having an effect on people who had been ill for a long time, and it seemed to be changing their attitudes to their illness. They were prepared to go off and try things when before they had been fatalistic. The conclusion was that the healer was spending time with them, empathising with them, and making them feel important. She was doing the things that good doctors do, but now find it so much harder to do in a few minutes.

On a more systematic basis, Dixon began offering his patients the chance of ten healing sessions. After the weekly sessions on Thursday mornings, the research team were amazed to find that as many as 80% of the patients felt better. More than half said they were 'much better' and stayed much better the next time they were asked three months later, even though – looked at under a microscope – the health issues still seemed to be there.

The research could not confirm whether this was the healer, or something else, which had a direct effect on their sickness. But it could, and did, draw conclusions about the crucial importance of time. There was a clear implication that taking regular time with patients matters a very great deal. The research was published in the *Journal of the Royal Society of Medicine*, and sceptical rage poured down on the heads of Dr Dixon and his team.

The point is not the use of Healers but that relationships in healthcare are vital, especially when you are isolated. Spending time with people, and building people into a wider social network where they feel valued and useful, is critical to people's recovery from ill-health – just as it is critical to staying well. Yet our healthcare systems are not well-organised to provide it. It was this gap that one innovative project in rural Cheshire tried to fill.

Ashworth Time Bank is a member of Timebanking UK and one of the most successful and active time banks in the UK, with over 400 members operating in 14 villages. Its members have made a huge success of linking time banking with healthcare, including providing people with therapists who can give them time.

"I say that being a time bank is like having an insurance policy," says Susan Ross-Turner, the time banks coordinator, "And you never know when you're going to need it."

Ashworth is now turning over about 200 'exchanges' a month. It has a holistic therapy group covering four villages and involving 30 complementary therapists, some of them giving time every week in return for training to upgrade their skills which the time bank organises.

Once again, this is about giving time and attention. "Some older people have not been 'touched' for years," says Susan, "and it is quite relaxing and at the same time emotional for them. They are lonely and this kind of therapy is given in a group first and then they can deliver it at their homes."

Ashworth has a link with homeless people and people on the substance abuse programme run by Turning Point in nearby Northwich, providing acupuncture three times a week. There is a prostate cancer group meeting three times a week, plus pilates classes and tai chi classes. There is an aquafit class, two 'keeping history alive' discussion groups and a textiles group for sewing. This is all run by a time bank that stays largely led by voluntary effort. It has a huge amount of health promotion activity and it is mutual.

So Susan jumped at the opportunity to get involved in the Timebanking UK research project to involve more formal health services, and in particular to link in the Parent and Carer Support (PACS) scheme which gives help and support for carers, especially of people who are terminally ill. Members of the scheme work alongside local Macmillan Nurses who had realised there was a requirement for a referral service for people who needed very informal support.

The local GPs were enthusiastic and supportive, but then came the surprise. Once the doctors were back in their consulting rooms, the referrals never came.

"I had hoped that the doctor would be able to prescribe time bank membership like they prescribe pills, but for some reason they were too busy. I was disappointed at first and now I don't expect any referrals to come," said Susan. "But I needn't have worried because the district nurses began to refer people in large numbers. It is extremely positive now and the phone rings all the time."

The PACS scheme also gets referrals increasingly from the local hospice when patients are sent home.

The lessons of Ashworth Time Bank, in this respect, are that the best way of providing a link between formal health services and informal mutual support is via the nurses who are genuinely on the front line. But it still raises some questions: why didn't the doctors get involved? Are they right not to, or are there sound reasons why they should? How do we integrate better and – behind all of that – the big question: do mutual support networks like time banks have a key role to play in the future of healthcare? This book seeks some answers.

Give and Take provides a background to this glimpse of the future – because Ashworth Time Bank reveals a view of public services where professionals, patients and the wider community have an equal, and a respected role in the health of their neighbourhood. It is the glimpse of a new kind of health service that understands the vital importance of social networks, and which does not have those obscure demarcation lines and administrative boundaries that can be so exhausting to navigate. So this is both a guide book to the role that timebanking might play in health in the future and an explanation of the findings of the Timebanking UK 'Resilience and Mutuality' active research project.

The project was commissioned by the Department of Health in the UK in 2012 to look at how much timebanking might provide a partial solution to three particularly difficult problems:

- The way that service provision is so fragmented.
- The ageing population with increasing needs, social and physical.
- How to implement the Health and Social Care Act, which was then newly on the statute book, with extra responsibilities for local commissioners – not just to tackle need but also to reduce it.

By October that year, Timebanking UK had drawn up a shortlist of the time banks and regions where they might best launch an experiment to target GPs and health services. They were:

- Warrington, Ashworth, Blackpool and Tameside (North West).
- Hull and East Riding (North East).
- Somersham and Colchester (East Anglia).
- West Sussex and Reading (South East).
- Lambeth, Tower Hamlets, Kensington & Chelsea and Camden (London).
- St Austell (South West).

Timebanking UK provided a wide range of places and types of projects, and deliberately so. By the end of 2013, when the project came to an end, it had involved 92 GPs across the places taking part, engaged 1,660 older people over 55 in timebanking activities and had seen almost 29,000 hours exchanged. In short, it had been a success.

In fact, timebanking had a good track record supporting health services already, and had done so since it began in the late 1980s. It had an excellent track record in reducing isolation, improving the health and well-being of older people and building stronger communities. These three objectives were at the heart of the project just as they are at the heart of this book. What the project tried to do, which had only been done fitfully before, was to involve the mainstream professions.

Here are some examples of what turned out to be possible:

- GPs writing 'prescriptions' for home visits where practical and emotional support is provided by time bank members who are fellow patients, and who themselves then visit the GP less frequently as a result of their participation.
- Community 'wellness classes' rewarding people with time credits for taking more control of their own health needs and support – from how to deal with an asthma attack, to detecting the first signs of depression.
- Self-help telephone support services by time bank members, using an assessment procedure designed by clinicians but operated by fellow patients, dramatically reducing the incidence of hospital admissions.
- A social network within a residential centre for women recovering from substance abuse, where training and support are provided by women for women, and 'paid' for in time credits through their own time bank.
- A rural time bank offering a 'health insurance' scheme under which all members are guaranteed two weeks' home support from other participants after an accident or illness.

These are all small ideas, carried out on a small scale, but they make a big difference to those involved, both as givers and receivers of these semi-formal services. The key question which lies behind them is this: what would public services be like, and health services in particular, if this kind of idea was mainstream and at the heart of the NHS?

This book tries to answer this. It goes beyond this particular project to look at the link between timebanking and health, what is possible now and what might be possible in the future, especially for the care of older people. It is, we hope, a way of looking at the future of public services as a whole – how they might be sustainable, human and people-centred in the future. And at the same time, how they can achieve an enormous step-change in effectiveness.

Background to a challenge

"Because of the shaking I don't go out a lot, but meeting others at the time bank has given me opportunities to meet people on a regular basis and do things together. We do knitting, have discussions and exchange ideas, and fundraise for projects. It keeps me active. It gives me personal pleasure to knit for others and see the joy it gives them. The time bank makes me feel better. I feel I am part of something, it helps me to cope and also forget the pain. I have made friends and if I need help I can call on them."

June, member of Rushey Green Time Bank, London, 2013

The concept now known as Timebanking stretches back to the early nineteenth century. These early experiments have inspired others to use time as currency to recognise the contributions people make to the greater common good or to hold together circles of informal volunteering, (notably the Tauschringe projects in Germany). Timebanking, as it is practised today in the UK, is a particular approach to rebuilding the social fabric, and it emerged from a psychological insight about people's need to feel themselves useful and the positive effect this can have on their health and well-being.

Since 1972, Betty Marver, at the Grace Hill Settlement in St Louis, USA, an independent network of health and human services, has pioneered new ways of enabling healthy productive lives. Central to many achievements has been the MORE time dollar project which uses a time-based currency to mobilises thousands of local people to co-produce health outcomes. They have inspired health related time banks across the world and informed theorists who have paved the way for this revolutionary pathway to increased participation and a reduced demand on health services.

The time dollar concept was further developed by a civil rights lawyer from Washington DC called Edgar Cahn. A heart attack at the age of 44 had left him in hospital experiencing the benefits of a good health insurance policy, waited on by nurses and doctors, he found himself wondering why he didn't enjoy it and realised that this was something that many, if not most, people in ill-health feel.

> People have a basic need to feel themselves useful, and constantly receiving and never being asked to give back can corrode people's lives.

It was 1980 and Cahn had worked alongside Sargent Shriver in Lyndon Johnson's War on Poverty. So in developing and promoting the system then called 'time dollars', he was responding partly to his experience in hospital and partly to the failures of American welfare to leverage permanent social and economic change. His central questions were asked in the USA but are relevant to the UK too: why do the social problems that the welfare state was designed to tackle recur generation after generation? Why is the support organisations give apparently so fleeting? Time banks were developed as a practical answer:

> "Help a neighbour and then, when you need it, a neighbour – most likely a different one – will help you. The system is based on equality: one hour of help means one time dollar, whether the task is grocery shopping or making out a tax return..."[1]

Early evaluation conducted by the University of Maryland's Centre on Ageing throughout the 1990s established that time banks were able to attract people who don't normally volunteer, keep old people healthier and cut the drop-out rates of volunteers.[2]

Most dramatically, the hospital group Sentara, in Richmond, Virginia, found that using a time bank to provide peer support for people with asthma, cut emergency admissions to hospital by 74% and saved $217,000 over two years.[3]

The Member to Member time dollar scheme run by a Health Maintenance Organisation (HMO) called Elderplan in New York City allowed volunteers to earn and pay time credits for giving and receiving non-medical services like, shopping, friendly visiting, bill-paying, hospital visiting, home repairs, walking clubs, support groups, self-help courses and others.[4] Mashi Blech, then Elderplan's director of community services said:

> "Often you can't buy what you really need. You can't hire a new best friend. You can't buy somebody you can talk to over the phone when you're worried about surgery. But by getting people helping through the time bank we want to involve people as co-producers of their own health care."[5]

Cahn's 1992 book *Time Dollars* also revealed some of the early frustrations of working with major service systems which were not yet ready to change.[6] But the basic system – more informal and more open-ended and flexible than a complementary currency – developed along similar lines in the UK and USA. It organises time credits as a new kind of currency which use time as a medium of exchange. Time-based currencies are tax free, and earning and spending them does not affect people's entitlements to state benefits. The systems have the following in common:

- One hour of help given to someone else earns one time credit.
- These time credits are deposited in the time bank.
- People can then draw out their time credits from the time bank and spend them on a range of skills and opportunities on offer from the other local participants.
- Everyone's contribution is welcomed and everyone's skills are valued equally – one hour earns one time credit regardless of the type of task.
- Details of all of the participants' skills, needs, availability and likes and dislikes are stored confidentially in the time bank computer.
- When they want a task done, participants contact the time bank coordinator, who acts as an intermediary and arranges for an appropriate participant to carry out the assignment.
- Computer software counts each transaction made between participants and issues people with regular statements.

How timebanking began in the UK

The story of timebanking in the UK started in 1996, when two social innovators visited the USA. David Boyle visited Edgar Cahn in Washington as part of a Winston Churchill Travelling Scholarship. Martin Simon visited the successful Maine Time Dollar Network in Portland and attended the first Time Dollar Congress. Both came back determined to bring the idea to the UK.

Boyle raised the money through the King's Fund to invite Cahn to speak at two UK conferences, one in London and one in Newcastle. He also went on the Libby Purves *Midweek* programme on BBC Radio 4, in October 1997 and made a huge impact. In the meantime, Martin Simon and Joy Robinson designed a Timebanking system for use in the UK and raised the money from the Barnwood House Trust to launch the Fair Shares network of time banks. As a result, the first UK time bank was launched in Stonehouse in Gloucestershire at the end of 1998.

Boyle was then an associate at the New Economics Foundation through which, and together with Sarah Burns and Dr Richard Byng, he was instrumental in launching the first time bank in a UK health setting, in the Rushey Green Group Practice in Catford.[7]

Fair Shares and the New Economics Foundation also worked in cooperation with two other innovative organisations, Valleys Kids in Wales and Gorbals Initiative in Scotland, to launch a national organisation that was then called Time Banks UK, (now Timebanking UK), which became a charitable trust in 2003 with offices in Gloucester. Timebanking UK remains the national umbrella organisation with a current membership of 300 time banks whose members have exchanged over 2 million time credits. This national network acts as a custodian of the knowledge and skills, undertakes research and training and pioneers new applications. It is a community of learning and the regional networks provide opportunities for collective reflection and an information democracy.

New software also makes it possible for time banks across the country to transfer time credits so that a member in London, for example, can earn time credits helping out in their local community and his or her mother living in Newcastle can use those time credits to 'buy in' the social support she needs from her local time bank.

Timebanking Wales, under the stewardship of Geoff Thomas, developed the idea of a 'token economy' utilising time credits that are printed as 'notes' and can be exchanged for access to learning, cultural and social activities. This has attracted major investment from the Welsh Assembly and from the European Commission, and this approach has contributed very successfully to improving social care in the former mining areas in the Welsh Valleys and beyond. The Garw Timecentre in Blaengarw, which began in 2004, is just one of their exemplary projects. Timebanking UK and Timebanking Wales share a rich history of collaboration and continue to work together to innovate, redefine and extend the reach of timebanking. Spice, a social enterprise, was set up in 2009 to take their time credits approach mainstream, under the leadership of Becky Booth and Tris Dyson.

That is the background to the idea of time banks. The questions at the heart of this book are around how much time banks provide a partial solution to some of the intractable health issues that face the NHS and UK society as a whole. The healthcare system here, and elsewhere – this is not unique to the UK – is beset by a series of interlocking challenges that threaten to raise their costs to an unsustainable level. These include the following:

An ageing population

By 2023 there will be more people aged over 50 years than there will be people aged under 50. This will put an enormous tax burden on the younger minority of the population, who will have to pay for a large part of the public services that will be needed by our ageing population. Not only are people living longer – average life expectancy by 2030 will almost certainly have risen above 85 – but people will also be more isolated. They are increasingly likely to be living alone. By 2021, over 30% of our households will be single person only.[8]

Modern lifestyles

The trouble is that many of the hidden ties that bind communities and families have been broken over the past

40 years. Two related changes have been shaping society. One is that we tend to do things alone, whether it is watching the television or participating in social media. The other is a growing lack of trust. Fewer than one in three people believe others can be trusted, which is down from 60% in the 1960s.[9]

Modern lifestyles mean that people move around far more and the make-up of the typical family is changing rapidly.

By 2050, many children will have no siblings or close relatives. We can no longer assume, therefore, that the informal care, freely given and worth billions of pounds if paid for in cash, will still be available to underpin the more specialised health care provided by professionals.

A typical family has 1.6 children, and the parents are increasingly likely to be unmarried, divorced or remarried.[10] There is a danger that, as people get older, they will sink into a prevailing culture of suspicion and increasing isolation.

Social limits to healthcare

The gap between rich and poor is continuing to widen and the health of the socially disadvantaged is still more at risk. Coronary heart disease is three times higher among unskilled men than among professionals, and that gap has widened sharply in the last 20 years. Further, stroke deaths in people born in the Caribbean and the Indian sub-continent are one-and-a-half times higher than for people born in this country – a differential that has persisted from the late 1970s.[11] Children up to the age of 15 years from unskilled families are five times more likely to die from unintentional injury than those from professional families.

Economics

There are various elements to this, but perhaps the most important – given its link to diabetes – is the impending obesity epidemic, which means that 10 million Britons could be diabetic by 2020, victims of bad diet and lack of exercise. If unchecked, the cost of obesity-related diabetes will swallow up health budgets. One in five adults are now classed as obese, along with one in nine children.

The 'baby boomer' generation is getting older and will continue their reforming march through our culture. They have changed sexual politics, the structure of the family and countless other cultural norms. They are bound to have an impact on the demand for health services and, if services do not expand accordingly, there will be a strong lobby for change from a generation that first exercised its political muscle in the 1960s.

Back in 2002, the Wanless Report concluded that an increase in understanding, self-help and engagement by the public in public health, over the next twenty years, would save the NHS £30 billion every year by the year 2022 – that was then half the current annual budget of the NHS.[12] This shift is only in the very earliest stages.

One organisation which has made a strategic effort to think about new directions is the innovation agency NESTA (National Endowment for Science, Technology and the Arts in the UK). NESTA's People-Powered Health project looked at how we might have missed the critical untapped resource – the users of the system, their families and neighbours. Conventional thinking suggests that this approach – from peer support to co-delivery – is fraught with dangers and compromise. Actual experience, as described in a series of films which the People-Powered Health team made, is that it can be transformative, changing the power balance between people and professionals.[13]

There is a huge untapped demand from patients and service users to use their time and human skills to help other people, as long as it is in some way mutual.

NESTA calculates that People-Powered Health along these lines will cut NHS costs by at least 7% and maybe up to a fifth.[14] Even 7% comes to £4.4 billion in England alone.

Their programme looked at innovations that had been developed over many years – from peer support networks to expert patient groups, doctors prescribing exercise to group consultations and to timebanking – and asked what would happen if these became a standard part of long term condition management. A people-powered health approach along these lines would:

- Mobilise people and recognise personal strengths as well as family, friends, communities and peer networks that can work alongside health professionals.
- Redefine the relationship between patients and healthcare professionals, focusing on the needs and aspirations of patients, but with both sides gaining more from the relationships.
- Blur the artificial boundaries between health, public health and social care, and between formal and informal support for patients.

Timebanking is one of the mechanisms promoted by the People Powered Health team because of its ability to involve people who never normally volunteer, including those who are usually the object of volunteering – and has a proven record of building up viable social networks and of strengthening communities.

The Resilience and Mutuality Active Research Project - funded by the Department of Health Third Sector Investment Fund (Excellence) and devised by Timebanking UK aimed to better prepare time banking to take a significant role in this people powered approach to health. A project coordinator worked closely with GP surgeries in 14 areas, helping them to work with communities and with older people to implement a more cooperative approach to prevention, treatment and recovery. Through the time banks local people would provide their own low level social care, watch out for the well-being of the more vulnerable among them and grow social capital. The plan was that a closer working relationship could evolve as GPs began to take on new responsibilities for commissioning.

By then, a number of time banks had been experimenting with recommendations by local doctors for patients to join the time bank, literally a prescription for social action, and had attracted hundreds of previously passive consumers of public services to become co-producers of care. The assumption was not that timebanking was the only way of achieving this, but as a pathway with a track record, that it should be taken seriously.

The project asked the following seven questions of health providers:[15]

- Do you ask your patients, users or participants what they enjoy doing for others?
- Do you look out for regular opportunities for them to help others?
- Do you welcome their involvement in the running of your organisation, and do you log the time that they work for you?
- Do you reward them for their cooperation?

- Do you ask them to pay back for the specialist services they receive from you, by giving more general help to others?
- Do you organise opportunities for mutual support between peers, either one-to-one or in groups?
- Do you participate in local events and community activities alongside your 'service users' and their families, friends and neighbours?

The following chapter explains some of the answers.

Time banks and health

"Individuals who were isolated, were
not members of a club or community
group, whose contacts with family and
friends were poorly developed, difficult
or non-existent, were between two
and three times more likely to die"

*George Kaplan, Jukka Salonen
and Richard Cohen, 1984*

One of the fascinating ways that timebanking can work is that some groups of NHS patients might suddenly provide solutions for another group of NHS patients, if the right barriers are broken down.

This is what has been happening in Warrington. The Warrington Voluntary Action time bank began in 2012 as an initiative by the local authority worried about social isolation among older people. The first time bank members were recruited by knocking on doors. Two years on, there is now a Silver Service Club, which provides a lunch for isolated older people and respite breaks for carers who need to go out. Everyone involved in running these services earned time credits for doing so.

"It is a very flexible form of volunteering," says Development Officer Philip Blocksidge. "We have been explaining it in terms of a kind of micro-volunteering. You can drop in and drop out."

The Silver Service idea originally came from another group of young people with moderate mental health needs who had been meeting at the Westy Community Centre. It was their idea that they could offer something in return. That's how it came about.

There is something revolutionary about this. It makes no sense to support old people without any reference to the needs of young people, or loneliness without any reference to the needs of those with mental health issues. Together, there is some potential synergy – they have complementary needs and abilities – but if you keep them completely separate it begins to limit the amount of mutual support that might be possible. So care becomes the exclusive preserve of professionals. Not so in this case: the patients have a purpose and a useful role which makes them feel good about themselves, and the isolated older people have a lunch club.

This is an important lesson for those introducing mutual support into health care systems: the moment you start where people are, with their needs and skills – you very rapidly find yourself working across professional boundaries.

Improving the health of older people

At the Rushey Green Time Bank, launched in a GP practice in Catford in South London in 1999, the idea was that doctors would refer patients to the time bank, either for help or because they needed involvement in group activity. It might have been very simple things, from help with shopping to a friendly voice over the telephone from someone who has been through the surgery before. Rushey Green has been evaluated twice, and both evaluations confirmed that it was effectively rebuilding social networks and could also make people feel better. They also demonstrated that the time bank was particularly beneficial for people with combined physical and mental symptoms.[16]

Another UK pioneer was the Fair Shares Community Time Bank in Gloucestershire which offered its participants a novel county wide 'health insurance' scheme called Rest Assured. All active members of the time bank were guaranteed that, should they have an accident or an unexpected stay in hospital, other participants would visit, do their shopping, run errands or whatever else might need doing for up to two weeks after their return to home.

In Glasgow, the Gorbals Time Bank ran a fresh food delivery service and a simple farmers' market, paid for in part with time credits. Vegetables were collected from the market by van and distributed across the community. The workers earned time credits and spent them across a whole range of opportunities open to them through the skills of other participants. A similar project was pioneered in Islington.

A recent evaluation was carried out at the Paxton Green Time Bank (PGTB), which is attached to an innovative group practice in Lambeth, by one of the doctors. Three quarters of the respondents said that joining the time bank had improved their quality of life (42% even said it had helped them save money), but the really interesting findings relate to people with depression:

- 76% agreed that PGTB helped to lift their mood.
- 68% agreed that PGTB had made them feel better about themselves.
- 67% agreed that PGTB had reduced their loneliness.

Out of the 21 survey participants who reported currently suffering from depression, 15 (71%) felt that the time bank had improved their depression symptoms. As many as 83% said the time bank had helped them make friends.[17] The study concluded that the time bank was making an impact on four key areas, all of which mattered to patients:

- Alleviating symptoms of depression and other chronic health problems.
- Making new friends in the community and reducing social isolation.
- Money-saving.
- Sharing and developing new skills.

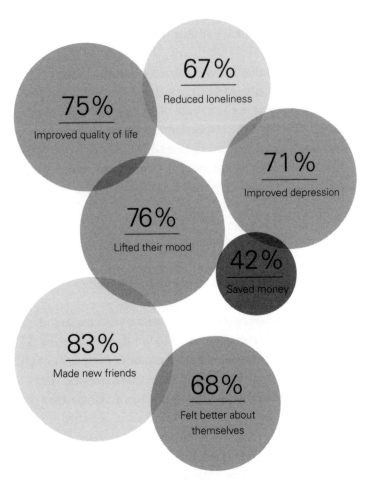

67%
Reduced loneliness

75%
Improved quality of life

71%
Improved depression

76%
Lifted their mood

42%
Saved money

83%
Made new friends

68%
Felt better about
themselves

KEY AREAS OF IMPACT

● Alleviating symptoms of
depression and other
chronic health problems.

● Making new friends in the community
and reducing social isolation.

● Money-saving.

Sharing and developing new skills.

Source: Paxton Green Time Bank Evaluation Survey

Like Paxton Green, Colchester Time Bank got off to a good start with the local surgery, which agreed to give them space to promote themselves, put them on the in-surgery TV system and welcomed 'time bank champions' regularly to the surgery.

They were soon also working with the local dementia care team and with the local authority youth service, helping them teach basic cookery skills to young people, another clear area where the skills that are needed are very widely available in the population.

Often it is learning new skills that keeps older people healthy, which is why West Euston Time Bank's sewing project was such a success.

Reducing isolation

One of the most substantial, consistent and neglected findings in all of medicine is that the presence of close and supportive family and friends protects and buffers us against the impact of disease. We know that lack of friends can be as dangerous to your health as smoking. Staying fit and well is easier when someone is there to encourage and support you, be it with caring words or with a sharp prod.

Time banks were not necessarily designed with this problem in mind, but they might as well have been. The idea, from the very start, was that this was not traditional volunteering, with all the overtones of *noblesse oblige.*

> By concentrating on what people can do and like doing for themselves and others, rather than on their presenting problem, the emphasis shifts from other forms of professional interventions that can inadvertently restrict people to a passive role.

Take Christine, for example. She had been unemployed for some time due to depression and health issues, and was referred to the Ashworth Time Bank. Her parents had both died shortly before. She had been their main carer and she had become lonely and isolated. Initially, she came to a coffee event at a member's home, and she spoke quietly, almost in a whisper and gave little eye contact.

It took some encouragement to get her along to the next events. But the time bank didn't give up and Christine came to one of their Sunday morning walks, and during the stroll she starting to open up and talk to other members. As they were all leaving, she said she had felt really down that morning when she woke up and wasn't going to join them, but was really glad she had made the effort. Christine turned up, unprompted now, at other events. One 75-year-old member noticed a poster for an 'Improve Your Memory Session' and told the group she would love to attend but, because of mobility problems and the venue being a good walk from the bus stop, she wouldn't be able too. Christine then offered to give her lifts to the group and said she would like to attend herself. The time bank set up the exchange, the two got on well and so the cycle continues.

Then there was Geoff (not his real name), 70. He was referred to the Help Direct Time Bank in Blackpool. He had recently been bereaved and needed support to reduce his social isolation following his wife's death. They had been married for 43 years. The issues he presented were isolation, loneliness and the emotional effects of bereavement, and the doctor very sensibly realised that this was not a problem that would be solved by his usual pharmacological armoury.

Geoff engaged with a local walking group through the time bank, attended a computer course through Age UK and a bereavement group at the Trinity Hospice. He was soon earning time credits through befriending and offering support to another older man who had also been bereaved. These two people have shown each other empathy and understanding, they have given peer support and reduced their feelings of isolation, while sharing coping strategies. A mutual solution and also a low cost one. Imagine the impact of such exchanges if everyone had access to a local time bank.

Timebanking UK shares a dream of a time bank in every doctor's surgery. Often reducing isolation is also about making a series of links with and between local organisations. As part of the research project, Hull and East Riding Time Bank made a connection with their Older Adult Mental Health and Dementia team, dovetailed with their Dementia Ambassador training. They involved the University of the Third Age (U3A) and the

East Riding Clinical Commissioning Group (CCG), as well as the Long Term Conditions Team. Most time banks maintain links with a range of local Agencies and look for opportunities to bring together the more informal self-help, arts, faith, sports, environmental, cultural and other socially-minded groups.

Building healthy communities

"We often see people who would dearly love to be a part of society again, after prolonged unemployment or sickness, but have nowhere to turn to achieve this," says Dr Saul Marmot at the pioneering health centre in Bromley-by-Bow. "The problem is often exacerbated by the pressure they feel to not be a 'burden on society'. It is often very difficult to be able to start filling in forms, applying for jobs and integrating back into a working environment. Some specific barriers to achieving this are low self-esteem, social isolation and a lack of experience. These barriers often seem so great, that people can't even take the first step."

That was why they set up their own time bank in 2012, because it could help build people's confidence in overcoming this kind of barrier, and also build their self-confidence and social skills. "The supportive, low-pressure environment helps people to work to a deadline and to feel proud of their achievements. This undoubtedly has a profound positive influence on their physical and mental well-being."

These factors all confirm the findings of a major review by the Corporation for National and Community Service in Washington DC, which gathered together 32 studies relating volunteering and health, and found that:[18]

- Volunteers suffering from chronic pain receive benefits from helping others even beyond what could be achieved with medical care. This included declines in the intensity and frequency of physical pain and also reductions in depression.
- Heart attack victims who volunteered afterwards reduced their risk of despair and depression, two factors that lead to mortality.
- Reduction in levels of depression for over-65s.
- Over-70s who volunteer 100 or more hours a year are a third less likely to die as people in a similar position who do not volunteer, and they are two thirds less likely to report bad health.
- Volunteering has a protective effect which lasts years after volunteering.

All the activities described above seem very varied, and they are often carried out through existing providers, the public and the voluntary sector. The role of the time banks is that they seem able to stitch these projects together, to reach deeper into the associational life of the community, to involve excluded groups and to add an element of mutuality – by changing the self-image of those who are usually the recipients of care, from feeling they are a burden, to being valued as contributors. They also provide a means by which service users with experience in the different professional 'silos' can help navigate each other across and around a system that continues to divide life into specialisms and departments with their own language and protocols.

This is the point where we need to explain a much misunderstood buzzword which illuminates some of the rich philosophy behind timebanking.

Co-production

The spark behind the 'co-production' idea emerged in Chicago. It was there that Elinor Ostrom, the 2009 Nobel prizewinner for economics, was asked by the Chicago police to tackle a confusing question for them: why was it that, when they took their police off the beat and into patrol cars – and gave them a whole range of hi-tech equipment that in theory could help them cover a larger area more effectively – did the crime rate go up?[19]

This problem is not confined to the police. It lies at the heart of why public services become less effective on the ground as they become less personal and more centralised. Elinor Ostrom's team decided that the reason was because that all-important link with the public was broken. When the police were in their cars and therefore unconnected with the everyday life playing out in their streets and villages, then the public seemed to feel that their intelligence, support, and help were no longer needed. Ostrom asked for a return to the sort of joint endeavour that once was at the heart of all professional work and called it 'co-production'.[20] It explains why doctors also need a reciprocal relationship with patients, why teachers need to find out how their pupils will learn best, and why politicians need the cooperation of the public, if they are going to succeed.

Chicago was also the city which Robert Sampson studied in the mid-1990s with his team from the Harvard School of Public Heath, trying to get to grips with the social factors behind violent crime. They split the city up into more than 900 different neighbourhoods and found, to their surprise, that none of the factors that are traditionally supposed to make a difference to crime – poverty for example – really seemed to be relevant. What did make a difference was what you might call a latent sense of co-production among people. It was whether they were prepared to intervene if they saw youngsters hanging about. Sampson called it 'collective efficacy'.[21] He described it as a "shared willingness of residents to intervene and social trust, a sense of engagement and ownership of public space".

At the heart of the concept of co-production, some decades later, are three very important linked ideas.

First, the realisation that professionals need their clients as much as the other way round. As the social critic Ivan Illich put it: "If you let institutions grow, become big and powerful through time, then these are the phases. While they're small they'll be relatively productive and as time and bureaucracy and power are assembled, they begin to become less and less productive. Then they'll begin to decline in productivity until they become counter-productive."

Second, the implication that service users and local people, who are sometimes seen to be a deadweight, a burden or source of irritation on an exhausted public service system, are also assets and are miserably wasted by the current system. They are a potential resource for providing the relationships and human skills and support which service systems can't provide, but which are enormously important for their effectiveness.

The third implication is the vital importance of a 'core economy', a term coined by the economist Neva Goodwin.[22] This is the notion that all local activity – parents bringing up children, looking after older people, or making neighbourhoods work – is not some magically inexhaustible resource outside the economic system. It is what makes the rest of the economy possible. So if we neglect this core economy or just allow it to be colonised by the market place, then we do so at our peril.

Those are the basic assumptions of the set of ideas called 'co-production' emerging on both sides of the

Atlantic. It is a slippery phrase, but it can broadly be defined as follows:

> "Co-production means *delivering* public services in an equal and reciprocal relationship between professionals, people using services, their families and their neighbours. Where activities are co-produced in this way, both services and neighbourhoods become far more effective agents of *change*."[23]

Communities need strengthening if they are to take up the co-production challenge. John McKnight and his colleagues at the Asset-Based Community Development Institute in Chicago have identified that six key elements are always present in every story of successful community building:

- The skills of local residents;
- The power of local associations;
- The resources of public, private and non-profit institutions;
- The physical resources and ecology of local places;
- The economic resources of local places;
- The stories and heritage of local places.

Time banks are fully fit for the purposes of providing a new local infrastructure for community building. Timebanking UK and Nurture Development[24] which are leading the training and development of Asset-Based Community Development (ABCD) in the UK, are working together. John McKnight and Edgar Cahn are both members of the stewardship group overseeing the development of ABCD Europe.

There remains a debate about whether time banks are best embedded in services or operating alongside them, hosted by voluntary organisations or communities. Time banks need to avoid being viewed as a separate voluntary organisation or as yet another project in need of external funding. They prosper when they are recognised as a tool for the promotion of reciprocity to be used to encourage participation – whether it is for the co-production of services, a route to community empowerment, a means of reviving and sustaining new kinds of social networks or for objectives we have not even thought of yet.

Time banks also suggest an answer to the welfare conundrum, that delivering services to people who are supposed to accept them gratefully and passively, which undermines their ability to resist life's difficulties, also fundamentally undermines their ability to be the heroes of their own lives. There is also something about reciprocal services, on the other hand, where we ask people for something back, and give them the respect that goes with being equal partners in delivery, which can turn that situation around.

One of the difficulties for those testing out reciprocal solutions is that they often seem to conflict with the way healthcare services themselves have been developed. They rely on face to face influence, when the trend has been a focus on virtual interactions from behind a screen.

They appeal to generalist, everyday skills that are in plentiful supply, when the trend has been toward increasingly scarce and expensive interventions by specialists. They are amateur, in the very best sense of the word, when the trend has been to overvalue efficiency and undervalue effectiveness. They rely on the idea that the users of services, and their families and neighbours, are a vast untapped resource, when the trend has been to regard them as clusters of needs and deficiencies. They focus on what is strong and what can be built on in local areas, when the trend has been to collect data on what is wrong or what is missing.

Co-production represents a different pattern for the future of healthcare. It represents an attempt to tap into the resources that are there in every community. It is an idea of services which are, as their basic purpose, hubs to make possible massive increases in active citizenship, mutual aid and voluntary activity, not through the voluntary sector but through a re-alignment of the public sector with the public. Human beings acting together can solve problems that nothing else can solve.

In recent years, health services have depended increasingly on three primary sources – government, commercial enterprises and voluntary organisations. A fourth source of health, that people have depended on for longer than they have on the first three put together, is community.

The time is right to bring it back and we must mainstream new methods for building stronger, sharing communities using powerful tools like timebanking. Without community, none of the other sources can ever be truly effective; with it, we might stand a chance of a healthy future together.

⊙ Findings

"They reach people that I can't find. And once
I can find them, that's when we can start
to get people engaged in the community,
and mixing with different people. And
that's why I love the time bank, because
it mixes completely random people."

*Time bank coordinator interviewed by Ruth Naughton-Doe
about their involvement in local time banks*

Ruth Naughton-Doe was seconded as a social policy
student to the South London and Maudsley NHS
Foundation Trust. She met Zoe Reed, Director of
Organisation and Community at the hospital, who had
been involved in timebanking from the start. Zoe sent
Ruth to Timebanking UK and to the New Economics
Foundation. So began her interest in how to measure the
success of time banks, which she pursued with a PhD that
is an evaluation of timebanking in the UK.

The result of the PhD was a tool which time banks
can use to evaluate their success. It also led to Ruth's own
involvement in Timebanking UK's Department of Health

research project during which she interviewed coordinators and GPs at three time banks in the north, south east England and central London.

She met one GP who signed his surgery up to the project because he felt there had been a surge of need in primary care, which would only get worse. He said there was a *"tsunami of need racing into primary care"*. His local time bank had presented to a conference for GPs on 'GP burn-out' which had been well attended. There was interest from the GPs in the region, including three surgeries signing up to hear more.[25]

The GPs were particularly interested in the role of timebanking in supporting patients with dementia. Dementia is a growing problem, and often it was hard to deliver positive news about it. Connecting people with the time bank was something GPs felt they could offer patients.

One time bank coordinator reported that GPs were helping her find 'hard to reach' time bank members, such as isolated and vulnerable older people. They knew where the people who most need the time bank were, and could connect them. For example, she told Ruth about one person referred to her by a nurse. The lady was only ever visited by the nurse, but knew nobody else. She would never have joined the time bank without the nurse, and would have remained hidden.

The time bank in the north of England had also been able to recruit some highly skilled members through the GP surgery. One time bank in London had set up a weekly social club group where members visited the surgery. When a member did not attend, the other members would go and check if they were OK. If a member went into hospital, the other members would go to visit them.

Difficulties

While there were many successes, there were also struggles. The first barrier was getting past the practice managers, who were often too busy or not interested enough to arrange meetings. Then, sometimes it was difficult to engage the GP surgery. Some GPs felt that, with the upheaval in the health service, people were reluctant to take on anything new. Job uncertainty, financial uncertainty and reform meant that general practice was reducing back to the bare essentials. This meant that time banks were needed more than ever, but it also meant the capacity to develop them was perceived to be lacking.

There was also the difficulty of actually collecting data. Despite many time banks agreeing to collect pre-test and post-test survey data there was a lack of coordinator time and the diversity of time bank aims, outputs and a lack of detailed record keeping undoubtedly made the evaluation of time banks very difficult (but there is a useful tool now available from the New Economics Foundation).[26] Ruth is also running a new service for Timebanking UK time banks to help with evaluation and impact assessment.

Promotional materials clearly need to be tailored to the local area. Getting a GP involved to help with promotion at local events certainly worked. Some training was also necessary – basic information about how to get into surgeries, but also information about how to deal with the type of members that come from the surgery. Time bank coordinators are going to be working with more vulnerable people, so they need to have the skills to deal with that.

Another important study that emerged out of the research project was an evaluation of the Salford Time Bank, which found that time banks gave isolated people credit for contacting other isolated people.[27] Salford Time Bank's Re-Energise project involved people to help them get fitter, but there was also a knock-on effect on diet: those who had taken part in Re-Energise had much healthier diets.

Beyond Salford, there is also evidence that people believe what they are told by peers and volunteers more than council employees or professionals.[28] There are also broader advantages in giving people a more active voluntary role in public services.[29]

Cost benefits

We have already seen that NESTA's 'People-Powered Health' project looked at how to apply the ideas behind co-production to long-term conditions – the most expensive, least successful aspect of NHS work.[30] NESTA's calculations, based on a range of studies, were that People-Powered Health along these lines could cut NHS costs by at least 7% and maybe up to a fifth.[31]

Evidence of other peer support programmes in the UK and abroad suggest that they give rise to savings in public costs of around £1 to £3 per pound invested, and more for the Health Champions volunteer programme which is closest to what is being proposed here, where there are savings in improved health and also in improvements in the lives and employment prospects of the champions themselves.[32]

The results of modelling the benefits of time banks, by a team led by Martin Knapp at the London School of Economics in partnership with Timebanking UK, found that the cost per time bank member averages less than £450 a year, but that the value of the economic and social benefits exceeded £1,300 per member.[33]

Peer support services in mental health are also extremely cost-efficient. The cost per day for one acute mental health hospital in-patient has been calculated to be £259; by comparison, the Leeds Survivor-Led Crisis Service successfully supports people at £180 per day."[34]

Informal solutions also come out well. Connected Care in Basildon has claimed impacts of over £1,000 per client, and a total of over £500,000 in savings across the town.[35] Savings in the Local Area Coordination project in Middlesbrough have been estimated at between £1.80 and £3 per £1 invested.[36]

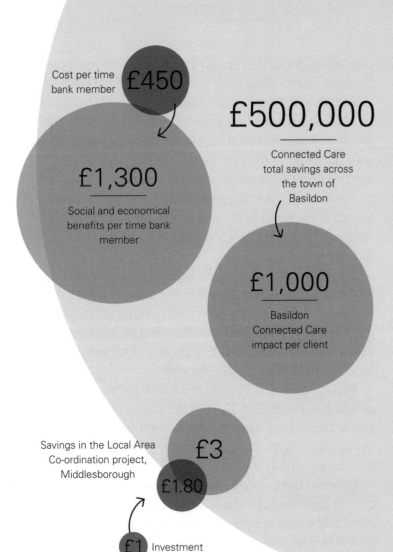

Cost per time bank member **£450**

£500,000
Connected Care total savings across the town of Basildon

£1,300
Social and economical benefits per time bank member

£1,000
Basildon Connected Care impact per client

Savings in the Local Area Co-ordination project, Middlesborough

£3

£1.80

£1 Investment

Source: Building community capacity: Making an economic case

Colchester Time Bank calculated, after just one incident, that they had potentially saved the NHS at least £2,000. One of their members was worried about a broken floorboard and a dud lightbulb on the landing. Another member fixed it and it may well have saved the taxpayer an ambulance call-out, a visit to A&E and a stay in hospital. If informal peer-support has proved itself so well, why does it remain a peculiarity, struggling for funding and outside the mainstream? Is it not possible to imagine a reform of public services that would use these ideas at scale?

Obstacles

The Resilience and Mutuality (R&M) project spent several months working on the 'blockers' to find out why it appeared so hard to mainstream innovative low cost programmes of valuable informal social support like timebanking in GP practices? It was clear that not enough GPs wanted to set them up, though many did want to take part in timebanking in some way. This was encouraging as successful time banks claim there is a clear need in the early days for a high level of enthusiasm from locally respected individuals, like GPs.

There are ways in which timebanking can seem to fly in the face of traditional medicine as it requires professionals to shift from being fixers of problems to catalysers of capacity.

Systems prefer quick-wins to long-term responses and – on the patient's side – there are cultural expectations that the NHS will provide, without individual users having to contribute anything more than their taxes. Other obstacles included:

- The short-term benefits of systems like timebanking are clear, but it is hard to find evidence of them morphing into longer term strategies.
- They need the right kind of staff.
- Institutions have to be able to let go of people's continuing relationships.
- There is the paradox of breaking boundaries yet also needing at least to have semi-permeable boundaries to get started.
- Welfare and philanthropic activity tends to impact on the short-term symptoms, not the underlying causes.
- It isn't immediately clear to managers that this is different from traditional volunteering.
- Mental health professionals in particular have ethical and data protection issues.
- If the project is too close to the local authority, it can also be stifling.

The R&M project looked at the ways in which these obstacles might be overcome, hosting workshops, discussions and consultations on the subject. They came to the following conclusions:

Recommendations

The cost cutting world is a mixture of help and hindrance to time banks

It is very important to keep a balanced view of the social drivers and the cost drivers if time banks are to be sustainable. Most people connected to time banks are not there to provide cheaper services for professionals, but people in the health system are having to find 'magic bullets' to reduce costs. This makes a meeting of minds difficult. At successful time banks the members define their own contributions and gains.

If people understand, as is likely, that their participation in timebanking will result in them drawing less on expensive health system services, then this has to be a benefit for the individual, the time bank, the health system and society.

Timebanking needs to refine and share how we all best sell to the medical community

Here are Colchester Time Bank's Top Tips for selling the idea to healthcare:

- Time bankers must focus their efforts to understand what each manager's role is and what issues they are trying to solve, then match the benefits of a time bank to their respective needs. It is often the number of these people agreeing that makes a success of the relationship with timebanking.

- Communications must be inclusive and use appropriate language.
- Communications must include stories, pictures of people, quotes and anecdotes.
- Provide evidence and measurement: many time banks do 'before and after' questionnaires to capture that information.
- Be clear about how much it costs to run a time bank.
- Develop your elevator pitch – key phrases include *supporting interventions with the elderly, people at risk or recovering from depression, reducing the 'heart sink consultation'* and *reducing prescription charges*.
- Know the latest legal and regulatory position and show how you can support the surgery's aims and objectives.
- Offer services that the time bank can deliver for the surgery – welcoming people, mailings, coffee events, spreading the word, administration, etc.
- Match what time banks can offer to their duty to the community – or Healthwatch, preventative health care agenda, or patient action groups.
- Let them know about your network and what you can bring about through collaboration – including stories and anecdotes.

- Make sure you establish both a common purpose and a clear delineation of roles, responsibilities and benefits.
- Peers – they listen best to other health professionals, so get a time bank opportunity at a medical forum rather than invite health professionals to a time bank if possible.
- Don't oversell – this is connected to understanding the long term and short term benefits and the relationship to costs and existing services as outlined above. Do not let surgeries think time banking is a magic bullet for health cost reduction and universally improved outcomes.

Funding safeguarding policy and action

In an increasingly litigious world, with high profile media risks, the medical fraternity is increasingly concerned about safeguarding. Insurance is available for time banks at special rates negotiated with a number of companies by Timebanking UK. It is also possible for host organisations that are already managing the safeguarding risk of their activities to incorporate the time bank without the need to invest extra money in insurance.

To make sure time bank members feel safe, references are taken up for all new members. By offering group activities, such as gardening or shared meals, time banks have been able to provide a safe space for people, like refugees, who are initially unable to provide references. The coordinator, as well as other participants, are able to get to know them better and relationships can be formed prior to references becoming available.

Timebanking UK has robust recommended safeguarding policies and procedures for members' time banks which have satisfied the insurance companies and ensure that time bank members feel as safe as possible.

⊜ What next?

"The health trainer suggested that I could cook my own meals instead of buying ready-made food and it would take my mind off my anxiety. It saves money and I've got more confidence now to find recipes on the internet and try them out."

Young mum, Salford Time Bank

If you have to get to an outpatient appointment at Lehigh Hospital, outside Philadelphia, then your chances of doing so without a car will often be nil. Buses are scarce creatures in this corner of Pennsylvania. There is a similar problem for patients who have been discharged, who don't have the luxury of a relative who can pick them up.

What do they do? The answer is that they often arrange for a lift through the local community exchange, and will be driven – not by ambulance drivers or other professionals – but by other patients, recovering ones or former ones. When you are feeling better, then you will be asked to do something similar for somebody else.

This is not the conventional way of doing things. There are some people who might refuse to countenance anything of the kind unless the drivers had undergone extra training and a full risk analysis. Other people might say – as they do say – that, if something's worth doing, then the government should do it. Yet there is something thrilling about the Lehigh way of doing things. The scheme saves money for the hospital, almost by definition, because people actually turn up for their treatment. But it also puts to work an absolutely huge human resource – people who are usually the recipients of public services, medicine or volunteering – and it turns out they are very good at it.

By 2010, the Lehigh Community Exchange had 450 members, run in the neighbourhood of Allentown by Kathy Perlow and her colleagues, and modelled originally on a similar project in Portland in Maine. It was funded, almost from the start, by the hospital. The trouble was, they never really used it. Nor did most of the medical profession, at least until the arrival of a new doctor in the area who could see the possibilities.

Abby Letcher came from Michigan, where she had been studying the social determinants of health. She was increasingly frustrated by the way the medical profession was failing to take them into account, "We know people need community, they need social networks and friends. That's why I'm a doctor," she said. "We don't have medicines for these things and, because of that, I was beginning to feel really useless."[37]

The prospect of being part of a new practice based on 'relationship-centred care' lured her to Lehigh Valley, and – when she heard about the community exchange – she was determined to build that in too. The medical side of the exchange is now coordinated through a new health centre called Caring Place, where Abby worked as a doctor, providing healthcare mainly for people in the area without health insurance, and looking for ways of building a healthier local community at the same time. Soon people were referred to the exchange if they had depression, and might feel better for helping other people. From there they didn't just drive other patients, they worked alongside nurses dealing with palliative care, providing a friendly face or a shoulder to cry on or a bit of shopping.

Sometimes they did it better than the nurses because they could provide things that professionals are unable to do, especially when isolation was the main problem their patients faced. "Caring individuals who are there because of you often do it better because they can provide a relationship," said Abby Letcher. "Of course there are paid professionals who care, but an informal support system will probably serve you better." This is how she explained it:

> "It is a fairly radical change, and it does challenge people's ethical and professional sense. But it has transformed the way we practice medicine. It has stopped us seeing our patients in terms of us and them, as if we were just service providers to people who are classed as 'needy'.

> We are no longer looking at them as bundles of need, but
> recognising that they can contribute, and when you see
> people light up when you ask them to do so, it changes
> your relationship with them. The culture has changed.
> The relationships are different, deeper and more
> therapeutic than they are in the usual doctor's office."

This is an example of how timebanking is able not just to improve the health of vulnerable people but to change the culture of the health delivery systems. There is a circularity about it: time banks find it hard to embed positive change in the structure unless the culture of those structures change, but – at the same time – the culture isn't going to change unless you go ahead and embed the time banks. It is the best argument for just getting on with things.

One of the reasons it's so hard to change the culture is that, in practice, the medical profession tends to ignore the social elements of ill-health – not because they don't accept them, but because the systems they work within find it so hard to work on them.

For service commissioners, there is evidence now that timebanking delivers real benefits across a number of agencies and communities. It is clearly not an alternative to good quality, accessible services, but it allows those services to be more effective. That is why Lambeth Clinical Commissioning Group (CCG) and the London Borough of Lambeth teamed up to deliver a programme to expand timebanking.[38]

How might timebanking develop?

Timebanking is a work in progress, even in health. The question is: how might it develop? The answer is that it would be worth looking at some of the ideas that developed during the short period of the time banking and health project.

Some of these are simple but effective innovations.

Westminster Time Bank was started alongside Westminster Carers' Service, but the 70 care professionals were sent elsewhere, leaving the time bank to facilitate much more mutual support. It wasn't until the coordinator Viola Etienne started talking to the members, in order to report back to their funders at the Big Lottery, that she discovered how effective it was.

"They said that it got them out of the home, whether it was to do yoga or learn English, if it wasn't their first language, it meant they could get out and get a bit of exercise," she says now. "We can't do professional respite care, but the time bank provides a space for the carers to support each other – doing befriending or phone support."

The point about the Westminster Carers' Time Bank is that it doesn't work as it was intended to, but it now provides a mutual network of self-help among carers. It can't provide respite care, but it can provide a great deal more – if carers can summon up the courage to ask. And helping other people out is paradoxically helpful to yourself.

"We are so used to people being *helped*, that we have to pretend there are all these things we can't do just to qualify for more help," says Viola. "The time bank doesn't work like that. If you can help someone else, you feel so much stronger yourself, and it makes it easier to ask next time you need something yourself."

So many of the time banks involved in the project were expected to be innovative. Colchester Time Bank approached Colchester Borough Homes, which manages the sheltered accommodation schemes, and joined up some of their staff as part of their employee volunteering scheme. They also approached and enlisted several volunteer drivers from the local community transport scheme. They were soon getting referrals from GP care advisers, community matrons and social workers, via the local social prescription initiative. Exchanges involving older people included teaching foreign languages, gardening, DIY, teaching IT skills, completing forms, companionship visits, knitting items to sell for charity, supporting a singing group, attending information workshops to pass to other older people, administration, teaching music and giving lifts.

All these time banks have been feeling their way towards what works best, and without any kind of national guidance or policies for the commissioners that might support their efforts.

One 2009 government study proposed a series of rights for peer support groups which might support mutual volunteering of this kind:[39]

- Use of commissioners' and providers' rooms and facilities for meetings.
- Opportunity to apply for local grant funding based on simple criteria like the number of members.
- Publicity by local services and on government websites.
- Automatic enrolment for patients, carers and service users (with an opt-out).
- Flexible working for staff who volunteer to run peer support groups.

Organised in the right way, this would also provide a whole new dimension to choice – an option to give and receive mutual support – as well as providing a cadre of volunteer navigators. It would also potentially unleash energy from public service users capable of underpinning the long term survival of services with a human face, and of broadening the scope of services that are provided. The new mutual support network would not take work from existing professionals or managers, but it would also be able to provide the kind of options that services ought to provide – befriending, advising, DIY eg changing light bulbs for older people – which they are currently unable to.

There are other national policy changes that might be needed so that these ideas can be brought to bear more widely, and these are covered in the next chapter.

It is possible to imagine how time banks might work if they were extended across the NHS. All patients, and especially older patients, could be joined up to their local time bank – probably by default, on an opt-out basis. Every patient being discharged from hospital could be told that a volunteer would come to see them at home, and go shopping for them if they needed it – and that they would be asked if they could play the same role later for somebody else.

Every Neighbourhood Watch group, every University of the Third Age (U3A) group and every day centre would include similar infrastructure, which would allow them to keep an eye out for lonely people in need of support.

The same kinds of systems would work in every public service outpost everywhere, and every surgery would have a cadre of patients who were providing advice, navigation, transport and a range of other services – organised through the public sector as a key part of their mission.

Technology

There are now over 30 software packages available for managing time bank exchanges and recording time credits. Timebanking UK provides software for members, initially this was through an in-house system called Time-On-Line, but last year a partnership was formed with hOur-World in the USA and their open source Time and Talents software is now available to all Timebanking UK members.

Rushey Green Time Bank tested the system over an extended period with their 1,000 plus members, operating from a Doctors' Surgery in south London. It allows members to detail requests, see where they are on a map and what services are available nearby, share news and events, post calendars, and create special interest groups with facilities to restrict or expand mail messages and SMS texts to specific groups and people.

But it's not all about technology - the presence of a central figure in the time bank to build loyalty and trust has also been identified as important in many of the time banks in the UK, Italy and Spain.[40]

This combination of human contact and advances in technology make it possible to replicate the collective memories that used to be present in all communities. The software knows who is available, with what skills and the people know who are likely to get on with each other.

❼ What we need to do

"It has given me a great boost and made a great difference to my life. Initially, I thought can't do anything, but staff helped me find what I could do and that gave me so much confidence."

Maggie, Argyll and Bute Timebanking

Since 1893, the Voluntary Nursing Service of New York (VNSNY)[41] has served vulnerable, at-risk, and chronically-ill populations in New York City. Every day it has over 35,000 patients and members in its care through a comprehensive range of short-term or post-acute, long-term and managed care programmes.

The VNSNY Community Connections TimeBank was one of the key programmes funded by VNSNY's community benefit fund.[42] Under the management of VNSNY, the time bank grew fast to a membership of over 3,000 people. Half of the members were non-English speaking so the timebank hired staff who were bilingual in English and Spanish and trilingual in English, Mandarin and Cantonese. Over 70% of members were born in another country and only 17% were white. Just over 40% were over 60 years old and only half had access to the internet. There were over 140 organisational partners and more than 180 business partners. Over 285,000 hours of service exchange have been recorded, though the actual total is significantly higher, with an estimated value of almost $3 million.[43]

While the members frequently expressed how participation helped reduce their isolation and made them feel better about themselves, a targeted study highlighted that even 80-year-old members believed their physical health was improving as a result of their membership. Those with the lowest self-reported annual income (under $9,800) and those who took the survey in Spanish reported the highest level of positive impact from time bank membership.

Other key findings from the VNSNY TimeBank's evaluation, a one-off survey of members, include:

- 48% reported improvements in self-rated physical health.
- 72% reported improvements in self-rated mental health.
- 73% of those with an annual income of less than $9,800 reported that membership helped them save money.
- 82% reported improved quality of life
- 93% reported that they are now exchanging with and befriending members of different ages, backgrounds and cultures.

- 79% reported that the time bank will help them to remain in their homes as they age.
- 67% reported increased access to health and other community services.
- 98% reported that, despite their advanced years, they are now able to use their skills to help others.

Many members reported experiencing shame on a daily basis, primarily because of their inability to communicate in English with others in their communities. VNSNY found that, for many members, joining the time bank and having the opportunity to share their skills increased their feelings of self-worth and made the members feel less ashamed and more accepted.

The idea of embedding a time bank in a healthcare setting clearly worked in New York City, and – although there are particular arrangements which are unique to that city (like the size of the operation) – it offers a model for testing elsewhere.

Policy directions

There are some key questions here. How might we go about embedding a network of time banks in the NHS, so that every patient has the opportunity to give back in some way to neighbours or fellow patients? And how might we encourage the proliferation of community time banks to enable citizens to take the lead on public health agendas and localised prevention strategies? Should we also consider what other knock-on effects of re-populating our health provision with unpaid co-workers made up of patients, their families and members of the local community?

In Baroness Julia Neuberger's book about older people, *Not Dead Yet*, she described how her uncle was neglected in three of the four hospitals in which he lived his final weeks.[44] She explained that the one exception was also the hospital which was the most cash-strapped:

> "When my uncle eventually died, in the hospital which really understood and respected his needs and treated him like a human being, there were volunteers everywhere. In contrast, there was barely a volunteer to be seen in the hospital which treated him like an object, although it was very well staffed. At a time when public services are becoming more technocratic, where the crucial relationships at the heart of their objective are increasingly discounted, volunteers can and do make all the difference."

Julia Neuberger was writing shortly after the first Mid-Staffordshire revelations. What she suggests is that citizens and volunteers are potential antidotes to this kind of abuse. In wards where older patients might otherwise be mis-treated or ignored the mere presence of ordinary people and volunteers are the eyes and ears that we need. Human beings provide that kind of alchemy, however target-driven the institution is around them.

Julia Neuberger was talking about hospitals, not about social care and companionship, but having people working and volunteering alongside professionals will help to remind them of what is important, to see situations through the eyes of an outsider; but they have to be *working* alongside, not just observing. Observers seem not to have the same effect: they are regarded as controls, not as fellow human beings.

This begins to make clear the outlines of a new objective in public services which can bring the power and energy of mutual support to bear on every area. It means an enormous revival of civic life, of citizenship and an extension of the concept of volunteering, (not through the voluntary sector – this is not about middle class semi-professionals ministering to the needy) – but through the public sector, where the beneficiaries support each other, as a major element of a new, more mutual, design.

A recent report for the CentreForum suggests that this would mean that every service outpost would include or involve some mechanism for allowing service users to become equal partners in the delivery of services – and capable of rebuilding social networks.[45] These networks would make up a new mutual infrastructure that supports people where they live and in informal or semi-informal ways. Our experience of timebanking shows us that, to succeed, this new infrastructure will need to be people-led, place-based, fuelled by reciprocity and meet with the average person's expectations around equality and fair play.

This is a policy direction towards restoring a culture of community. To achieve this professional health care providers and commissioners must:

- Find ways of resourcing communities directly, so that they can become strong enough to sit at the table with professionals to plan a mutually supportive way forward, perhaps out of the savings they make possible in prevention.
- Involve the existing social networks and the informal groups, clubs and associations.
- Impact on life as it is lived, rather than operating within the artificial boundaries that have been set up between the various government departments.
- Do no more harm to the re-emergence of a culture of community.

Public and professional awareness of community development and peer support is still low, funding is insecure and far too bureaucratic, despite a demand for mutual support among patients. Traditional performance management systems also ignore their importance.[46]

Here are some policy considerations drawn from our first-hand experience in the field and from the work of the CentreForum.[47]

Developing the infrastructure

Experience suggests that the infrastructure will not just appear by itself. Connected, caring communities do not just happen and, given all the distractions of modern lifestyles, it is surprising that so many people still respond positively if they are asked to get involved.

People are assets but they need change agents like time banks to connect them with one another again. Research efforts are thankfully shifting from analysing needs to mapping assets. Simply knowing that an asset, like the skills of local people, exists gets you nowhere. Each asset has to be connected and activated. Only then will any productive action for change begin, any results be achieved, any power gained.

Local authorities will need to be facilitators and among their tasks will be to see what mutual support infrastructure already exists – and where they might encourage more to begin. The fastest way that time banks spread, as they did so rapidly during the last decade, was where local authorities and health services held themselves back from setting them up themselves. Instead, they identified and funded respected voluntary organisations or community groups to host local time banks, serving neighbourhoods of up to 4,000 or so people.

There has often been a middle manager within the sponsoring agency who has driven things forward from behind the scenes. Development officers who can seek out enthusiasts and encourage them have been successfully employed, converting a general interest in the concept into a set up group of people willing to commit a few hours a week for twelve months to share the task. Doctor's surgeries are still the most appropriate settings for time banks. People still trust their doctors. The direct pay back for Doctors would also be considerable when you consider that there are still 57 million GP consultations a year for minor ailments at a total cost to the NHS of £2 billion, which takes up, on average, an hour a day for every GP[48].

Change the requirements for public sector contractors

This approach implies that every bid for a public service contract will be expected to include answers to the following questions:

- How do you plan to help rebuild social networks?
- How do you plan to encourage mutual support among users?
- How do you plan to reduce the level of need for your service year by year?

This is important for other reasons too, because – as things stand – the most powerful inducements on contractors are to increase the level of need, not reduce it. This is an important shift towards achieving a more preventive service too, but it will also encourage innovative thinking about how to create the kind of social networks around services that we are trying to achieve.

Often what the contractors will do is link up with and fund a time bank, or similar local project, to help plug their service into a network of mutual support. That is the main way by which this supportive infrastructure is going to be funded – by contractors who need to explain to commissioners how they will fulfil their obligations to encourage mutual support among their users and the wider community.

ƒ

This is how the experience gained in the Resilience and Mutuality Action Research Project described in this book might be given a nationwide infrastructure in health and social care. It would provide an extra dimension to health-care, and an extra responsibility for patients and anyone under the NHS umbrella and within public health, but it is a dimension that will transform the rest by default.

An NHS with a time banking dimension would be broader in what it can achieve, more flexible and more human for patients and their families. The evidence also suggests, coincidentally, that it would be more cost-effective.

Appendix 1
About Timebanking UK

Timebanking UK is the only national umbrella charity linking and supporting time banks across the country by providing inspiration, guidance and practical help. Time banks link people locally to share their time and skills. Each member's time is equal: one hour of your time earns you one time credit to spend when you need.

There are over 35,000 people sharing their skills among the member time banks of Timebanking UK and they have generated over 2.3 million hours of mutual support. There are new time banks being set up every week. With the twin drivers of the need for more self-reliance caused by the public deficit crisis and the current government's commitment to hand more power and responsibility to local communities and citizens, the political climate could not be more conducive to time banking.

Timebanking UK supports all models of timebanking in both urban and rural settings. Organisational time-banking, where organisations join and share resources in the same way, is also becoming a central feature of the long term sustainability of our networks across the country. These models also share the five core values of Timebanking UK:

- **People are assets**
  The real wealth of this society is its people. Every human being can be a builder and contributor. A time bank recognises this by allowing members to define for themselves what they consider to be a valuable asset and enshrining its value through the hour for an hour principle.

- **Redefining work**
  Work must be redefined to include whatever it takes to raise healthy children, preserve families, make neighbourhoods safe and vibrant, care for the frail and vulnerable, redress injustice and make democracy work. A time bank provides liquidity to activity that informally contributes towards these and other essential elements of a civil society.

- **Reciprocity**
  The impulse to give back is universal. Wherever possible, we must replace one-way acts of largesse in whatever form with two-way transactions. 'You need me' becomes 'we need each other' at a time bank.

- **Social capital**
  People need a social infrastructure. It is as essential to them as roads, bridges and utility lines. Social

networks require investments of social capital generated by trust, reciprocity, and civic engagement. A time
bank creates a system that builds social capital – every
action leaves a footprint.

- **Respect**
  By respecting and recognising value in the contribution
  that every individual can make, we hard-wire a positive
  and critical feedback loop into all aspects of our work.

Future plans

The central idea of timebanking is that everyone can have
all they need for their own well-being by contributing what
they can to building and sustaining a healthy community life,
caring for the marginalised, bringing up children to flourish
and by fighting injustice. Everyone has a role to play. That
means Timebanking UK is committed to the following:

Supporting time banks to continue to develop and thrive as social innovators

Central to achieving our mission is the continued development of a range of time banks across the UK – in public
services, at community level, and between organisations.
The greater the number of time banks, the more transfer-
able the currency becomes and the more sustainable time

banking can become. That requires a sustained and reciprocal relationship with member time banks. Member time banks are the source of practical grassroots credibility upon which Timebanking UK has underpinned its objectives. We are committed to co-producing our work with member time banks and listening to their national voice.

Building the appetite for and understanding of timebanking

Alongside our aim of building the infrastructure around timebanking is an equally important strand that focuses on building understanding of timebanking and co-production at a strategic level. A system change agenda is supported by the recognition that those in the field who are trying to work in new ways are working counter to some of the structures already in place. This objective therefore represents Timebanking UK's efforts to examine the barriers that exist to working in new ways, so that commissioners understand the full implications of co-production and timebanking. It means we:

- Facilitate and provide training and development solutions in timebanking and co-production, working with place-shaping and local strategic bodies, such as local authorities. We co-design and co-produce a range of training solutions to grow a practical understanding of timebanking.

- Conduct research into new applications and implications of time banking and co-production. Working with partners we explore ways to overcome barriers, evaluate the impact of timebanking, and research new applications of timebanking, disseminating findings through publications and active social media campaigns.

Be a learning organisation

We need to be able to reinvest the learning generated by grass roots experience. Timebanking UK harvests this learning to build a compelling case for system change and sustains an in-house environment that is hospitable to our members. In that sense, our other two strategic objectives are interlinked – the practical, on the ground wisdom of time banks is the fuel that supports the learning, development and research workstreams of the rest. In the same way, the more an understanding of timebanking grows through learning, development and research, the more we can gather ongoing evidence.

Growing and supporting a thriving membership of time banks

The grassroots innovation, expertise and effectiveness of member time banks provides Timebanking UK with the evidence needed and legitimacy required to push a national scale agenda around timebanking and co-production. It is therefore essential that we invest in supporting existing members, listen to their national voice, making sure their time banks can be as effective as possible in bringing about a system change agenda.

Underpinning this is our aim to see as many time banks as possible develop and flourish as part of connected regional social marketplaces. We are therefore working to grow the membership by:

- Working alongside major public service organisations to seed time banks into their mainstream service delivery, making sure wherever possible that their services are co-produced.
- Working with communities to make sure that timebanking is an easy to use tool for communities and groups to mobilise and organise themselves along lines of equality and social justice.

These different applications of timebanking become stronger when they are linked together, as part of connected regional marketplaces. We therefore facilitate the building of regional networks and hubs of time banks, so that the sharing of local expertise, best practice and capacity amongst regional members is part of the membership package.

Developing the membership package

We are building our online community of practice which houses a bank of best practice, guidance and case studies, start up materials, videos, newsletters and policies and procedures. We are working on creating a basic networking functionality especially for time bank brokers and co-ordinators. Our membership packages are tailored to suit the organisation involved and include:

- Structured consultancy, training and support at various levels:
    i. remote and on-site training, guidance and toolkits for setting up time banks and their different applications, working on both strategic and operational development plans.
    ii. specialist expertise on fundraising, marketing and insurance, as well as in thematic areas like young people, criminal justice and social care.
    iii. facilitation support for building regional hubs and networks of time banks utilising mentors / buddies and our Associate Consultants on a day to day level on-site.
- A quality scheme and the opportunity to achieve accreditation.
- Connections – brokered relationships between time banks that share particular interests or audiences, and with funders, commissioners and

providers with the opportunity to be part of both a regional and national network of time banks.

- Events – regional learning and social events for the practitioner community to exchange ideas and experience and build a shared sense of identity.
- Resources – free of charge software, mobile phone app, start up materials, publicity and promotional literature.

Equipping the profession of timebanking

We expect the number of time banks to grow dramatically. In order to ensure that this period of growth is sustainable, it is essential that there exists a critical mass of people who are trained in timebanking and understand what co-production means in practice. We want time banks to receive accredited qualifications or use of our quality mark and to help build the capacity of local time banks to deliver effectively through work placement schemes. We also want a growing number of people who understand the practical implications of time banking and co-production, and put their skills to use for social good.

Investing in platforms for connected timebanking

Timebanking UK believes that whatever form time banks take, whether embedded in a community or a housing association, they are more sustainable when they are connected to a network of other time banks, and in particular, when they have access to a wide range of resources of the kind that organisations can provide.

In practice, this could be anything from tickets to a football match to access to a spare meeting room or the use of a minibus. The greater the pool of resources that is available to people, the greater their scope for enterprising social initiatives. 'Small' time banks become 'big' by being part of a wider network linking resources that are underused by the market economy from across the public, private and community sectors. Equitable access through a time bank allows individuals and groups, who might traditionally be excluded from access to a pool of resources beyond their reach, to use the market in a creative and dynamic manner.

Member time banks can all benefit from a platform for organisational resource sharing being more readily available. At the moment Time-On-Line can handle the online exchange of thousands of hours of support every day, but it is built for an audience of individuals sharing time and skills, as opposed to organisational members sharing resource in a time economy. For that reason, Timebanking UK has formed an exclusive partnership with hOurworld in the USA to roll out a new piece of software for the UK.

Time and Talents software enables time bank members to use the software to post offers and requests, to arrange exchanges (overseen by a coordinator) and to feedback on their experiences. It enables time banks to search for resources and skills by theme and geographically to enable a more fluid interaction with other time banks locally, regionally, nationally and now internationally. There is also a mobile phone App which opens up a world of opportunities for people who will be able to access timebanking while 'on the move'.

Training and development solutions

Redefining the value relationships that exist between commissioners, providers and users of services to bring about co-production is a change management process of epic magnitude. For that reason, it is important for Timebanking UK to influence the way in which professionals and policy officials are trained. We are working with existing training organisations, such as the The National Council for Voluntary Organisations (NCVO), who train a cadre of voluntary sector leaders, to build a comprehensive understanding of co-production and time banking into the curricula, and build a set of programmes and events in this field.

Conducting research into new applications of time banking and co-production

Despite the enormous growth in timebanking over the past ten years, and the explosion of interest at present, it remains a relatively young and unexplored concept. Member time banks are constantly innovating, pushing the understanding of how and where timebanking can be applied. From co-producing adult social care services, through to exploring ownership models where commissioners, providers and users have an equal stake in co-produced services, there is a vast range of areas ripe for more comprehensive analysis.

Timebanking UK wants to be able to explore major thematic and topical research questions around time banking and co-production, bringing them to a wider audience. As host to many hundreds of active time banks, Timebanking UK has access to a range of expert witnesses. With research partners, we can explore live research questions and bring findings to a wider audience through publications and events.

In the short term, Timebanking UK has identified four priority areas for research:

- Exploring how member–member time banks can form a major part of adult social care solutions.
- Evaluating the impact of timebanking – developing appropriate tools for measuring the contribution towards a civic GDP.
- Exploring how time banks can be financially sustainable.
- Exploring mutual ownership models for time banks that involve commissioners, providers and users having equitable stakes.

Contact details

Timebanking UK
The Exchange, Brick Row
Stroud GL5 1DF
www.timebanking.org
01453 750952
info@timebanks.co.uk

Other useful contacts

Timebanking Wales
www.timebankingwales.org.uk

Volunteer Now Northern Ireland
www.volunteernow.co.uk

Volunteer Development Scotland
www.volunteerscotland.net

New Economics Foundation
www.neweconomics.org

Co-production Network
www.coproductionnetwork.com

Asset-Based Community Development
www.abcdinstitute.org

❷ Notes

1   E Cahn and J Rowe, *Time Dollars*, Philadelphia: Rodale Press, 1992
2   Time Dollar Institute, *Angels and Health: The use of time dollars in the healthcare industry*, Washington: Time Dollar Institute, 2000
3   See note 2
4   Metropolitan Jewish Health System, *An Evaluation of Elderplan's Time Dollar Model*, New York: Metropolitan Jewish Health System, 2003
5   Quoted in D Boyle, *Funny Money: In search of alternative cash*, London: HarperCollins, 1999
6   See note 1
7   See www.rgtb.org.uk
8   E Evans and J Saxton, *Five Key Trends and their Influence on the Voluntary Sector*, London: nfpSynergy, 2003
9   D Halpern, *Social Capital*, Bristol: Polity Press, 2003
10 See note 8
11 Neighbourhood Renewal Unit, *Health and Neighbourhood Renewal*, London: Department of Health, 2002
12 D Wanless, *Securing Our Future Health*, London: HM Treasury, 2002
13 See http://vimeo.com/63558665
14 See http://www.nesta.org.uk/publications/business-case-people-powered-health
15 M Simon: *Your Money or Your Life: Time for Both*; Freedom Favours & Timebanking UK, 2010. See http://www.freedomfavours.com
16 See for example T Harris and T Craig (2004): *Evaluation of the Rushey Green Time Bank: Final report to the King's Fund*, London: Socio-Medical Research Group, St Thomas' Hospital, 2004
17 V Virani and the Paxton Green Group Practice, *Evaluation of Health and Wellbeing Benefits of the Paxton Green Time Bank (PGTB) Service*, London: PGTB, 2014
18 http://www.nationalservice.gov/impact-our-nation/research-and-reports#HBR

19 E Ostrom and W H Baugh, *Community Organization and the Provision of Police Services*, Beverly Hills: Sage, 1973

20 R B Parks, P C Baker, L Kiser, R Oakserson, E Ostrom, V Ostrom and S L Percy (1981), 'Consumers as co-producers of public services: Some economic and institutional considerations', *Policy Studies Journal*, **9**, 7, 1981, 1001–1011

21 R J Sampson, S Raudenbush and F Earls, 'Neighbourhoods and violent crime: a multi-level study of Collective Efficacy', *Science*, **277**, 1997, 918–824

22 N Goodwin, J A Nelson, F Ackerman and T Weisskopf (2003), *Microeconomics in Context*, New York: Houghton Mifflin, 2003

23 D Boyle and M Harris *The Challenge of Co-production*. London: NESTA, 2009

24 Nurture Development – see website: http://www.nurturedevelopment.org

25 R Naughton-Doe. Unpublished PhD research, University of Bristol.

26 This is called *No Small Change*, available at: http://www.b.3cdn.net/nefou ndation/6e006679e8a6d649fd_3num6frei.pdf
This is best-practice in current evaluation. There are also useful tools available through TBUK based on Ruth Naughton-Doe's PhD research

27 NHS Salford, *Time Banking Interim Report*, Salford: Hall Aitken, 2011

28 See for example B C Sloane and C G Zimmer, 'The power of peer health education', *Journal of American College Health*, **41**, 2011, 241–245; and K Milburn, 'A critical review of peer education with young people with special reference to sexual health', *Health Education Research*, 10, 1995, 407–420

29 Department of Health (2006), *National Evaluation of the Pilot Phase of the Expert Patient Programme*, London: The Stationery Office

30 http://www.nesta.org.uk/areas_of_work/public_services_lab/health_and_ageing/people_powered_health

31 NESTA, *The Business Case for People-Powered Health*, London: NESTA, 2013

32 N Hex and S Tatlock, *Altogether Better Social Return on Investment Case Studies*. York: York Health Economics Consortium, 2011

33 M Knapp. A Bauer, M Perkins and T Snell *Building Community Capacity: Making an economic case*. Canterbury, London and Manchester: Personal Social Services Research Unit (PSSRU), 2010. See: http://www.pssru.ac.uk/pdf/dp2772.pdf

34 T Basset, A Faulkner, J Repper and E Stamou, et al (2010) *Lived Experience Leading the Way: Peer support in mental health*, London: Together UK, 2010

35 A Bauer, J-L Fernandez, M Knapp and B Anigbogu, *Economic Evaluation of an 'Experts by Experience' Model in Basildon District*, London: LSE Health and Social Care, 2011

36 Peter Fletcher Associates, *Evaluation of Local Area Coordination in Middlesbrough*, Northumberland: PFA Ltd, 2011

37 The interview with Abby Fletcher was carried out in 2009. See also: J Lasker, L Baldasari, T Bealer and E Kramer, *Building Community Ties and Individual Well Being: A case study of the Community Exchange organization*, Lehigh University, PA, 2006, available at www.lehigh.edu

38 http://www.lambethcollaborative.org.uk

39 M Horne and T Shirley, *Co-production in Public Services: A new partnership with citizens*, London: Cabinet Office, 2009

40 http://www.is.jrc.ec.europa.eu/pages/documents/ICT4EMPL TimebanksBoyleforwebsite.pdf

41 In August, 2014, ArchCare, the healthcare ministry of the Archdiocese of NY, acquired the TimeBank in its entirety as VNSNY is undergoing a major reorganisation and could no longer sponsor it.

42 This account draws from the case study published on the site given in note 39

43 *New York*, 23–30 December, 2003

44 J Neuberger, *Not Dead Yet, A manifesto for old age*, London: HarperCollins, 2008

45 D Boyle, *Turbo-charging Volunteering*, London: CentreForum, 2014

46 See for example D Boyle, A Coote, C Sherwood and J Slay, *Right Here, Right Now: Getting co-production into the mainstream*, London: NESTA / New Economics Foundation, 2010

47 See note 43

48 See Selfcare Forum http://www.selfcareforum.org

✪ Acknowledgements

The authors would like to acknowledge the invaluable input and advice, both here and during the project, from Ruth Naughton-Doe and Martin Simon.

Grateful thanks also to the time banks, time bank coordinators and time bankers whose efforts and imagination have made all this possible.

❷ Index